# Eliminate

# Plantar Fasciitis

# Pain in 3 Days

Seem too good to be true?

I probably wouldn't have believed it either.

Except that it happened to me.

And, it can happen to you too!"

Susan Dumas

Kaytek Consulting Inc.
Waterloo, ON,
Canada N2L5Y6
contactkaytek@gmail.com

## Disclaimer

No responsibility is accepted for the use of this information. Use the information presented in this publication entirely at your own risk. Neither the author nor Kaytek Consulting Inc. assumes any liability to persons for any loss, damage, injury, cost or expense incurred by any person using or relying on the information.

# Table of Contents

Disclaimer ................................................................ 3

Table of Contents ................................................. 5

Introduction ......................................................... 7

Chapter 1 – She'll Be Right ................................. 11

Chapter 2 – What is Plantar Fasciitis? ................. 15

Chapter 3 – What You Need to Stop Doing Right Now
.............................................................................. 23

Chapter 4 – What You Need to Start Doing Right Now
.............................................................................. 25

Chapter 5 – Be Wary of These Treatments           49

Chapter 6 – The First Attack ............................... 55

Chapter 7 – The Unthinkable Happens – Second Attack............................................................61

Into the Future with Happy Feet..............................67

Dedication.............................................................69

Resources.............................................................71

# Introduction

We take our health for granted not appreciating our bodies when they are healthy. Then something happens. It may be minor like a paper cut on an index finger. We might respond with ouch or darn at the time. Later, when we floss our teeth, all of a sudden we notice the discomfort of that cut with the dental floss wrapped tightly around our finger.

Generally, our feet don't get much attention. My husband says feet are like tires. They both get us around. We provide minimum maintenance for both by filling our tires with air, washing our feet and clipping our toenails. Then we're off to more interesting things. It's only when something goes wrong, like a flat tire that gets our full attention. Plantar fasciitis has the same effect on our feet. We can no longer keep motoring along until some repairs are carried out. Unfortunately, unlike tires which can be replaced, our feet must last a lifetime.

I'd never had any problems with my feet beyond a blister or stubbed toe. My first attack of plantar fasciitis brought an abrupt appreciation of what I had lost – the ability to walk comfortably. I call it an attack as it happened without warning and with considerable pain. It was the equivalent of driving over a nail causing my tire to go flat.

Plantar fasciitis was new to me. I'd never heard of it and could barely pronounce it. Surprisingly, I found little information about it and often discovered the information I was given by so called experts was useless for me and sometimes incorrect or incomplete.

Within this e-book I'll give you the information I've discovered since my first attack of plantar fasciitis in May 2003. I'll tell you what has worked for me and what hasn't. And I'll include some solutions I've uncovered but haven't tried. As everyone is different, certain solutions may appeal to you more than others. At least, you'll be informed and can make your own decision.

Most importantly, I'll reveal to you what gave me relief within three days when I suffered my second plantar fasciitis attack. At the time, I thought this was just another piece of information I'd missed. The speed of eliminating the pain was so startling I was compelled to research it further. So I searched the internet. I read the pleas for help, the questions and responses, the comments and suggestions in several online forums discussing plantar fasciitis. There was no mention of it. Why not? For some unknown reason, this information was not getting out.

My hope is that you will be better informed than I was. That you will also find quick relief from the technique I used to heal my plantar fasciitis injury. And that you'll soon be back on your pain free feet enjoying the activities you love.

# Chapter 1 – She'll Be Right

Although my first experience with plantar fasciitis was an acute pain in my foot, I thought it was just a severe cramp. It was painful getting going in the mornings, those first few steps out of bed, but not so bad if I kept moving.

I was in denial that anything serious was wrong with my foot. I believed 'she'll be right'. For those not familiar with the Australian lingo, she'll be right is a wonderful Australian expression meaning everything will be ok. However, it wasn't.

I hobbled around for over a week before accepting the fact that my foot was not healing. It was not just a bad cramp. It was time for a visit to my medical doctor.

Believe it or not, even the second time I had a plantar fasciitis injury, I was in denial. You'd think I'd learn. ☺

As you're reading this book, you've probably accepted the fact that you have a painful foot and are seeking relief. That's good. You need to acknowledge the problem and then you can start to find the healing solutions that work for you.

Be aware of any negative thinking you may have. For instance, replaying how your injury happened and blaming yourself especially if it was sports related. Dwelling on the cause and reviewing 'what if' scenarios is not productive.

At times, when we are in pain and nothing we try seems to be working to relieve the pain or working fast enough, we start to believe we'll never get better. Our desire is to return to the activities we were able to do without pain whether a fitness workout, a sport, a hobby or just walking comfortably.

Now is the time to focus on behaviors that will contribute to your healing. Take 30 seconds to do this visualization exercise and speed your healing.

- Close your eyes and take a couple of deep breathes.

- Picture yourself doing an activity you enjoy without pain such as a dance fit routine, playing a sport, hiking, or enjoying a leisurely walk on a sunny afternoon.

- Say out loud whatever activity you are doing and that you are doing it without pain. For example, I'm walking free of pain with my dog in the park.

You can repeat this visualization daily. A good time is just before going to bed to let it sink into the subconscious mind.

Bottom line, mindset is important. Even if you've suffered for a long time and think nothing is going to work, have faith and believe you'll be walking again without discomfort.

# Chapter 2 – What is Plantar Fasciitis?

Plantar fasciitis (pronounced fash-ee-EYE-tis) is one of the most common and least understood foot problems. Finding out what plantar fasciitis is helped me understand what was happening with my foot. It's the same when I take my car in for servicing. I always want to know what the problem was and how it was resolved.

First some background information on the foot. A foot contains 26 bones, 33 joints, and 112 ligaments. Together, our feet account for a quarter of all the bones in our body. Our feet are our body's foundation allowing us to maintain balance, body alignment, and the flexibility to move gracefully. A problem with our feet can affect our legs, knees, hips, pelvis, and spine.

The arches of the foot support the weight of the body for shock absorption and propulsion. The arches help us adapt to uneven surfaces. The fasciae provide strength to the arch and help stabilize the foot. Each step exerts considerable pressure over a relatively small area even if you have large feet. Over a lifetime, the feet are the brunt of the most wear and tear of any body part. Thus, our feet are more prone to injury yet often receive minimal attention.

Plantar fasciitis affects the arch and heel. Since this is the part of the foot acting as the shock absorber, it is easy to understand why it generates so much discomfort and pain.

Plantar refers to the bottom of the foot. Fasciitis is an inflammation of the fascia which is a band of connective tissue that stretches along the bottom of the foot from the heel to the toes forming

Plantar Fascia

Area of Pain from Plantar Fasciitis

Heel Bone

**Bottom of Foot**

the arch. The inflammation causes the tissue to become red, swollen and sore.

During the day the plantar fasciae (plural for fascia), stretch out with walking, etc. Then at night when we are at rest, they contract. So when you get up in the morning and take that first step, the shortened plantar fasciae generate the pain as you stretch them out.

The inflammation of plantar fasciitis is usually caused by the fasciae pulling away from where it is attached to the heel bone. When we are at rest, it begins to reattach to the heel bone. Then, when we become active again, it is torn away causing the foot pain.

The pain may be felt in the arch or closer to the heel where the fasciae attach. There can be a strong almost burning sensation on the bottom of the foot. In severe cases, the heel can be visibly swollen. Some people experience foot cramps while sleeping.

The heel pain is often confused with heel spurs. However, heel spurs do not cause pain. They develop in an attempt to relieve the discomfort from plantar fasciitis. The fasciae are pulling away from the heel bone so in response, the heel bone starts to grow in the direction of the fasciae. This extension of the bone is known as a heel spur. The good news is that heel spurs often resolve themselves once the plantar fasciitis has healed.

## What causes plantar fasciitis?

You may already know what caused your specific plantar fasciitis injury especially if it was sports related. I just stood up at my desk and tried to take a step. It felt like something snapped in my foot causing pain and an extreme cramp. I now know it was the fasciae tearing likely caused by a gradual build up of stress on my foot.

I'm listing the common causes so you can hopefully avoid future occurrences. About 10% of the population suffers from plantar fasciitis at some time during their life.

Causes of Plantar Fasciitis

- You are more likely to be affected by plantar fasciitis if you are a dancer, a runner, do step aerobics, or participate in sports like squash or tennis which require a lot of side to side lateral motion.

- A sudden turn putting excessive pressure on the bottom of the foot.

- Not completely stretching to warm up before participating in a sport or fitness activity.

- Your occupation can be a source of problems if you're on your feet all day or have a job requiring you to twist your feet e.g. lumberjack or hydro worker when they still climbed poles before they used lift buckets.

- Wearing improper footwear which doesn't support the arch of the foot properly e.g. flat sandals or thongs.

- Wearing shoes with very stiff soles – no flexibility.

- You'll be more vulnerable if your feet normally roll inward when you walk or run.

- Having a particularly high arch makes you more susceptible especially if your feet are rather rigid.

- Flat feet can also predispose you to plantar fasciitis.

- Being overweight puts more stress on the feet. Among plantar fasciitis sufferers, the majority are overweight. Seriously consider reducing your weight. Even a few pounds will help.

- As we age, the plantar fascia loses its elasticity. This causes excess strain where it attaches to the heel bone.

## When will I be better?

Now that we know what plantar fasciitis is and what causes it, the next question is - 'How long until I'm healed?' Unfortunately, this is a tough question to answer. Everyone is somewhat different and the level of injury varies as well. It also depends on how quickly you recognized the problem and started treatment. In my research in the forums, I found some people that were doing well after a few weeks, most seemed to take from several months to a year or two to be fully healed. I heard of one case that was unresolved after twelve years.

It was a year and a half after my first attack of plantar fasciitis before I could jump out of bed in the morning completely without pain. I was thrilled to be almost totally without discomfort three days after a treatment that resolved my second injury. I'm writing this in hopes that the same treatment can greatly shorten your healing time.

## Chapter 3 – What You Need to Stop Doing Right Now

There are two parts to treating plantar fasciitis. One is reducing the inflammation; the other is dealing with the original cause. You want to prevent further injury and reduce any activity which further aggravates your plantar fascia.

Stop

- Reduce or stop any sport or physical activity that caused the plantar fasciitis injury. I realize this is difficult if this is part of your job. Try to avoid any activity which would aggravate the foot further.

- Avoid lifting heavy objects as this places additional strain on the arch.

- This is not the time to do anything requiring you to climb a ladder. Those rungs can really hurt.

- Avoid going barefoot. You need good arch support. My injury happened in the spring. So that summer, I couldn't walk barefoot on the beach without pain. Watching others play beach volleyball made me shudder as the players stretched, jumped, and twisted their feet. Ouch! My foot hurt just watching.

- Avoid flat footwear with little support. Even if it is summer, you can find sandals with good support or just wear your running shoes.

- Avoid strengthening exercises until you are healed. Stretching exercises are acceptable. More on those later.

# Chapter 4 – What You Need to Start Doing Right Now

The most important item you need is a good fitting pair of running shoes to support the arch of your foot and the sides of your foot to avoid twisting of the foot. Although there are general guidelines for choosing a good shoe, it will help to know your foot type and the best shoe for it. There are three basic categories of feet: normal, high arched, and flat. Not sure of your foot type? Here's how to determine your foot type.

Wet both feet. Stand up straight with your weight evenly distributed on both feet. Then step on a dark, smooth towel or medium colored piece of construction paper to make an impression of your foot. Compare the shape to the following diagrams to determine your foot type. You may find your feet are slightly different or you are in between types. For example, you may have a slightly higher arch than the normal foot but not as high as the high-arched foot.

## Normal Foot

With a normal foot, you can see most of the foot with narrowing for the arch. This type of foot is biomechanically efficient for walking. When you walk, your weight falls on the outer side of your heel, rolls onto the outside of your foot slightly, then rolls inward to sag a bit in the arch area before pushing off with the ball of your foot and the big toe.

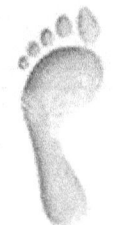

The normal foot needs a shoe with moderate stability and motion control, nothing too firm or too flexible, and good arch support.

## High-Arched Foot

If part of the arch is missing from your foot impression, you have a high-arched foot. When you walk, more of your body weight rolls to the outer side of the foot. So this foot shape doesn't absorb the shock of walking effectively. This places additional pressure on the bones, tendons, and ligaments of the foot on that side which can cause knee and lower leg problems.

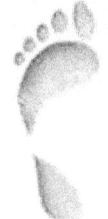

To compensate for the lack of shock absorption, shoes with ample cushioning and plenty of flexibility are best.

## Flat Foot

If you have flat feet, almost your entire foot will appear in the impression including all of the arch area. A flat foot is the opposite of a high-arched foot. So the opposite happens when you walk. Your body weight rolls excessively inward flattening the arch. Again, the weight of the body is not properly absorbed. This can result in even more problems to the hip, leg, shin, knee and lower back.

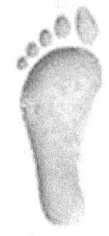

Look for a shoe that will help to control the motion of rolling inward. One with maximum stability, good arch support, and a heel that cups your heel to reduce motion is best. A shoe with a wide flared heel will provide support and help to reduce fatigue.

**Tips for selecting good running shoes:**

The shoes you choose don't have to be expensive as long as they meet the following general criteria taking into account your foot type.

- Go shoe shopping later in the day. Feet tend to swell as the day progresses.

- Avoid buying your shoes online unless you have purchased the exact same shoe before and fairly recently. Any small change to the shoe in style or materials may compromise the fit for your foot. Personally, I try on every shoe.

- Always try on several sizes close to the size you usually take. Try a half size bigger and smaller. Feet change with seasons and age. Sizes can vary by manufacturer.

- Try on different widths of the same size.

- Make sure you try on both shoes. Your feet can vary slightly in size with one foot longer or wider than the other. Always buy a pair that fits the larger foot. You can add an insole to the shoe for the smaller foot.

- Check that the shoes are the same size. Once I found a pair of shoes I liked that was the last pair in the store. When I tried them on, I discovered they were two different sizes! I still wonder if the person that bought the other unmatched pair was aware of the two sizes.

- Ensure you stand if you are having your feet measured as the toes spread while standing.

- Take along the socks or hosiery you will normally be wearing with the shoe.

- You may need a half size larger if you are wearing arch support inserts. Try the shoes on with the supports in them. Same advice if you are using heel cups or pads. Keep trying on half size larger shoes until you find a pair that is definitely too big. Go back to the next half size smaller. That may be the best size for you.

- The shoes should have sufficient arch support. Ensure the sides of the shoe are strong enough to hold your foot firmly while supporting the arch. To test this, roll your foot side to side with the shoe on. If you can go over on to the side of the foot easily, the shoe is too soft. If you can't move your foot much at all, the shoe is likely too rigid.

- Lace up both shoes and check for comfort on the top of the foot. Foot height can be overlooked. You may be able to adjust the tension of the laces and the number of eyelets used to get a comfortable fit. Otherwise, try on a different style.

- Ensure you tie your laces snuggly but not overly tight. Leaving them undone or too loose compromises the support your foot needs.

- Lace up from the farthest down eyelet pulling the lace snug to evenly distribute the tension. A crisscross or zigzag pattern is best.

- The ball of your foot should fit comfortably in the widest part of shoe. The shoe should be flexible enough that it bends easily at the ball of the foot. You can't walk in stiff shoes. It's like wearing planks.

- Check the range of motion the shoe permits. Avoid a shoe that allows too much side to side motion or twisting of the foot.

- The heel of the shoe should fit snugly and firmly without allowing your heel to slide up and down.

- Ensure there is about a finger's width of space between your longest toe and the end of the shoe. You should be able to easily wiggle your toes.

- Look for firm, cushioned support with some give.

- Check the shoes for ridges on the bottom, sides and top that may be uncomfortable for your foot.

- Check for good quality stitching and materials.

- Take the shoes for a walk on a hard surface.

- If the salesperson suggests the shoe will be more comfortable once it's broken in, shop elsewhere. A good fitting shoe should feel good right away.

- Consider buying a second pair to wear in the house. Most slippers don't provide enough support.

Over a lifetime, we take enough steps to circle the globe 5 times. That's equivalent to 115,000 miles. Good fitting shoes are essential.

This brings me to another topic – when to replace worn shoes.

Wearing worn shoes past their useful life can increase fatigue and cause foot and leg problems. If the sole is noticeably worn, likely the arch support is also worn out and not absorbing the shock of walking as effectively. You may notice more side to side foot movement as there is additional give in the sides of the shoes.

You may think your shoes are fine. Here's a quick way to check heel wear. Place your shoes on a counter or table. Bend over so you are at eye level with the heels. Check for wear and wear patterns. If you tend to place more weight on the inside or outside of the foot, that side will be more worn. If there is a definite angle, it's time to replace the shoes.

You know when the tread on your vehicle tires is low, that it's time to purchase new tires. It's much the same with your shoes. On average, you may have to replace a pair of shoes you wear regularly ever six months. If you are overweight, you'll need to replace your shoes more often.

In my mid-twenties, I had a pair of low heels I wore often to work. I realized they were getting worn but wasn't ready to give them up. One day I arrived home from work and walked into the bedroom to change my clothes. I collapsed onto the floor. My legs just gave out. It seems my legs had been compensating for the worn shoes to the point of exhaustion. That was the last time I wore those shoes. I had no further problems after giving them up.

**More things to start doing now:**

- Purchase some inexpensive arch supports. They make walking more bearable as they reduce the stretch of the foot by supporting the arch. I'm not recommending custom made orthotics. Just the type you can pick up at a pharmacy or discount store like Walmart. The first pair I purchased at a specialty foot store cost $75. The ones I bought at the drug store and discount stores were priced between $4 and $19. There are various styles with some having more support than others. They come in sizes for men and women. They are firm but made of a soft flexible material. Some are gel pads. You may need to try a few to see what works for you and at this price it is more affordable to do so. I still put arch supports in most of my shoes to prevent further injury.

- Standing barefoot in the shower can be painful. Try wearing a plastic or rubber sandal that has some arch support. These are the ones that are slightly shaped and conform to your foot. Avoid the perfectly flat ones.

- Icing the area near the base of the heel may help. The inflamed area is fairly small where the fascia attaches to the heel. So avoid icing the entire foot. Fully icing the foot causes the arch fascia to contract further when your goal is to stretch and relax them. Icing the whole foot will increase the pain when you try to put weight on your foot. To reduce the inflammation, use a small ice pack wrapped in a towel just in the heel area for no longer than 15 minutes. If you don't have a small ice pack, you can freeze water in a plastic bottle. Remember to leave room in the bottle for the water to expand when it freezes.

- Massaging the foot and arch gently may help relax the fasciae so they stretch out a bit thereby reducing any discomfort.

- Consider swimming as an activity. You can get a workout and stay off your feet. Try to keep a supportive sandal near the edge of the pool when you get out. Walking on cement and tile can be difficult.

- Another way to get a workout and stay off your feet, is riding a stationary bicycle. You get a good aerobic workout and retain the strength in your legs.

- Keep moving. This sounds contrary. You want your foot to heal. You're avoiding the sports you enjoy. And now I'm recommending you keep moving! The idea is gentle movement. Staying off your feet as much as possible allows the fasciae to contract as they do when you're sleeping. You want them to stretch. After you've been idle for awhile, lying or sitting down, do some stretches before standing up. This will help to alleviate the pain from those first few steps.

Following are some foot stretching exercises. You don't have to do them all. Try them out and choose what you prefer. One may work much better for you than the others.

Point and Flex Toe Curl

This stretches your arches to lengthen them and reduces the discomfort when you stand up. It also helps to lengthen the calf muscles. Do this exercise before you get out of bed in the morning to help reduce discomfort. You can also do this when you've been sitting for an extended period of time to stretch your feet before standing up.

- In a sitting position, straighten your legs keeping your heels resting on the floor.

- Point your toes and curl your toes under and hold for 10-20 seconds.

- Then slowly flex your foot up bending at the ankle and curling your toes up to a fully flexed position. Hold again for 10-20 seconds.

- Then relax for a few seconds and repeat.

- Do a set of 3 to 5.

## Ball Massage

- In a sitting position, roll your foot over a tennis ball or any ball about the same size. Ensure you are rolling the ball under the arch to stretch it.

- Avoid the painful heel area where rolling the ball may aggravate the inflammation.

- Apply enough pressure to feel the tight muscles but not so much as to cause pain.

- Roll the ball as far forward as you can and as far backward.

- Ensure you cover the entire width of the foot.

- Do this for two to three minutes for each foot to get a good stretch.

Towel Curls

- In a sitting position, place a towel on the floor. Ensure it is slightly crumpled so you'll be able to grab it with your toes.

- Using your injured foot, curl your toes on top of the towel pulling it towards you.

- Repeat 10 times.

- As it gets easier, increase the resistance by using a heavier towel or placing a weight on the end of the towel.

## Help your feet by reducing your weight

As mentioned previously, if you are overweight, consider reducing. There are so many reasons to slim down. At least once a week our local news station has a segment on a health issue that is either caused by excess weight or that weight has contributed to it. Excess weight does increase the stress on our knees, legs and feet. Even a small reduction in weight helps.

I know everyone says to lose weight. Not all have a good suggestion on how to accomplish weighing less. So I want to include some information on a couple of weight reduction systems that are sensible and work. How can I be so sure? It's working for me.

In the last few years I've discovered that many of the weight loss systems are based on eating foods that are low on the glycemic index of foods. The glycemic index measures the speed at which your body breaks down carbohydrates and converts them to glucose which your body uses for energy. Some carbohydrates break down into glucose in the digestive system at a slow and steady rate. This keeps us feeling full longer. Others break down quickly causing a glucose spike like eating a chocolate bar. It perks us up for a while. Then in a short time we're hungry again.

Some foods that are high on the glycemic index and should be avoided are surprising. I thought eating melons would be good but that is not the case. I thought pasta would have to be avoided. However there are some you can eat. Generally whole wheat or vegetable based pastas cooked to a la dente are acceptable.

The glycemic index was developed by Dr. David Jenkins, a professor of nutritional sciences at the University of Toronto, when he was researching the effects of carbohydrates on blood sugar for diabetics.

One of the best eating plans based on the glycemic index is the G.I. Diet by Rick Gallop. Rick Gallop was the president and CEO of the Heart and Stroke Foundation of Ontario, Canada. At the time, he wanted to lose twenty pounds. He tried the diets popular at the time such as the low fat, high carbohydrate diet. Nothing worked. He did considerable research eventually learning of Dr. Jenkins work. He tried the low glycemic index way of eating and lost the weight.

He introduced a few friends to it but they found it difficult to follow. So, Rick developed a simple method of categorizing food by red, yellow and green like traffic lights. The red light foods are high on the glycemic index scale and should be avoided. The yellow light foods can be eaten occasionally. You can eat as much as you like, within reason, of the green light foods. It's an easy to follow system and you never have to feel hungry. All his books provide a list of foods in each category and offer some eating plans and recipes.

There are several books in the G.I. Diet series. Some of the titles are:

- The G.I. Diet: the Easy, Healthy Way to

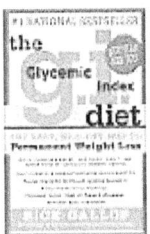

  Permanent Weight Loss

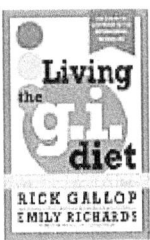

- Living the G.I. Diet

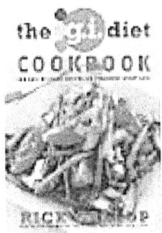

- The G.I. Diet Cookbook

- The G.I. Diet Express for Busy People

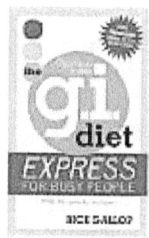

They are widely available worldwide and in many languages.

If you are interested in reducing your weight, I encourage you to try eating the glycemic index way.

Another terrific eating plan is presented by Jorge Cruise in the 3-Hour Diet. The idea is to eat a reasonably sized meal or snack every 3 hours so your metabolism stays at its peak and your body never switches to starvation mode and fat storing. Best of all, you can eat all your favorite foods – just in moderation.

The 3-Hour Diet book explains the program and why it works including a 28 day guide, the best foods to select and testimonials from those who have been successful following the 3 hour plan. Jorge also has a cookbook of quick to prepare meals for breakfast, lunch, dinner, snacks and desserts.

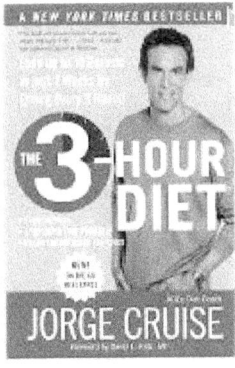 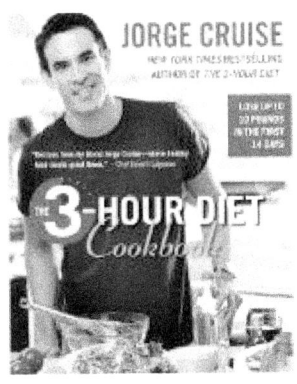

# Chapter 5 – Be Wary of These

## Treatments

Some of the following treatments are fine short term but have side effects. Others I have tried with poor results and, in some cases, increased my discomfort. Others I discovered while doing research and have no personal experience with them. I've included them to provide you with as much information as possible. You may have additional problems with your feet beyond plantar fasciitis or your gait requires the services of a foot specialist. In any case, use the following treatments with caution.

- If you have a great deal of ongoing pain, you can take anti-inflammatory drugs for a short time. These drugs have side effects over the long term. They provide some relief but are not addressing the real problem. However, they may be helpful short term if your injury was traumatic e.g. from an accident or a fall from a fair height.

- Using a heel cup was the first thing recommended by my doctor. A heel cup is made of hard plastic. It's placed in the heel of your shoe. The idea is to raise the heel up to take some pressure off the heel. But it does nothing for arch support and can cause stress in other areas of the foot. It didn't help me at all. The only people it may help are those with tight calf muscles. By the way, you need to buy two, one for each foot. A key piece of information I wasn't told.

- Heel pads have a similar function to heel cups. They are made of foam rubber, can be cut to any shape, and sometimes have a hole in the center to keep pressure away from a heel spur. Like heel cups, no arch support is provided.

- Cortisone injections. I understand these are quite painful. They appear to relieve the pain for some time until the cortisone wears off. This is similar to taking anti-inflammatory drugs. The pain is gone temporarily but the basic problem has not been dealt with.

- Custom orthotics may be appropriate if your plantar fasciitis is caused by how you walk – the flexing and rolling of your foot. You would need to see a foot specialist to diagnose this and they would provide a solution. A hard plastic material is often used for custom orthotics. The idea is to push up on your arch. Often this actually increases the pain. They are also quite expensive. I recommend first trying the softer arch supports readily available at pharmacies.

- Foot taping to hold up the arch and restrict movement of the foot is another option I've found. I haven't tried this. There seem to be a number of different taping methods. They require someone else to do the taping for you as you can't get the correct angles and degree of tightness on your own. It seems to be an acquired skill.

- If a medical practitioner recommends surgery, get a second opinion. Often the surgery is done to release the arch ligament or fascia. In my research, I found a number of cases where people had surgery, sometimes several times for the same plantar fasciitis injury. In most cases, it didn't resolve the problem. Generally, surgery is not necessary for plantar fasciitis.

- This next suggestion I have not tried personally. I've seen many advertisements for them on the internet. People who have tried them and discussed them in forums have had mixed results. What am I talking about? Night splints. The idea behind night splints is to keep the plantar fasciae stretched out while you sleep to avoid the pain experienced with those first few steps in the morning. This seems a reasonable idea. The splint is a foot and arch brace that wraps around the lower calf and foot to keep the foot flexed at 90 degrees as if you were standing. Cost ranges from $25 to $90. I've read mixed reviews of these in the forums. Some found a splint helpful others ripped them off after a couple of hours as they felt restrictive and uncomfortable.

- Along the same idea as the night splint is the night sock. This is an apparently more comfortable brace. It looks like a sock with a strap that stretches from the top of the sock to the toes. It keeps the toes curled up maintaining a stretch for the fasciae.

## Chapter 6 – The First Attack

It was a wonderful spring morning in May 2003. I had just finished a good workout at the fitness club and arrived at the office. It was time for coffee. I stood up at my desk and as I took a step, felt a sharp pain in the arch of my left foot. I stood there in pain for several minutes until I was able to hobble away completely unaware of the seriousness of my injury. I thought it was a severe cramp. That it would ease off soon and be back to normal. But that was not to be the case.

Several days later, my left foot was still painful, especially first thing in the morning. Those first steps getting out of bed were excruciating. I began to get up and hop to the bathroom. I found that as the day progressed, the pain subsided until I'd been sitting for awhile. Then it would hurt again when I tried to walk. So I'd limp along until I could gradually take a more normal step again.

After a couple of weeks of little improvement, I decided it was time to see my medical doctor. He diagnosed me with plantar fasciitis, something I had never heard of and could barely pronounce. He recommended getting a heel cup to raise my heel up and reduce some of the pressure. He directed me to the experts at a sports footwear shop to purchase the heel cup.

I have a small, narrow foot wearing a 5 ½ or 6 AA shoe. At the sports footwear shop, I asked if heel cups came in different sizes. The assistant wasn't sure. So he hunted through a barrel of heel cups (Yes a barrel! They must be big sellers.). He concluded that one size fits all. So I bought one. Yes, only one as only my left foot was in pain.

If you've had the pleasure of wearing heel cups you know that you need two, one for each foot, otherwise you limp as one heel is higher than the other. Neither the doctor nor the sports footwear expert informed me that I needed two heel cups. Yes, I spent the next few weeks limping. ☺

I expected to be better after wearing the heel cup for three weeks but I wasn't seeing any change. The doctor hadn't indicated any length of time for healing. I just assumed three weeks should be long enough. So, I called his office to make another appointment. His nurse practitioner suggested I go to the foot clinic.

The foot clinic was quite helpful. It was at this point I discovered I should have been wearing two heel cups. They checked my feet, watched my gait as I walked, and sold me a pair of arch support inserts for my shoes for $75. I felt lucky that I didn't need custom made orthotics costing several hundred dollars. Years ago, my mother had tried custom orthotics several times and found them hard and more painful than the problem they were to correct.

The foot clinic told me to expect a healing period of 3 to 5 months. I was shocked by the length of time. Yet, it would actually be much longer.

The foot clinic recommended I wear running shoes as much as possible. By now it was mid summer, the time of year I normally wear sandals. I had a pair of beach shoes that had a slight arch support that helped when I went to the swimming pool. However, I limped getting in and out of the pool but the swimming was good exercise replacing some of the walks I once took.

Interestingly, just before my injury, footwear rules at the office changed. No longer was wearing running shoes to the office allowed. I had to get special consideration to wear my running shoes. The runners did feel better even though they didn't look very stylish with my summer dresses.

Although I was wearing my running shoes at work, I didn't want to wear them around the house all the time. So, I needed another pair of arch supports for my slippers. There were also a few events where I wanted to wear dress shoes or sandals. I took a chance and bought more arch supports of various kinds and sizes at drug stores, Walmart, Zellers, etc. These ranged in price from $4 to $19. Amazingly, they worked just as well as the $75 pair.

Basically, this was all I did to heal my plantar fasciitis injury. No one mentioned stretching or icing or drugs to reduce the inflammation or the other gadgets to help alleviate the morning pain. A year and a half later I could hop out of bed in the morning without any foot pain. Yes, 18 months instead of the estimated 3 to 5 months.

Even after my plantar fasciitis injury healed, I continued to wear arch supports in shoes, boots, slippers, and some sandals. I never wanted to go through another plantar fasciitis injury again.

Now, when I buy shoes or sandals, I look for those with good arch support. I avoid thongs, flat sandals, and hard inflexible soles. I rarely go barefoot except at the beach. I always try shoes on with my inserts to ensure a proper fit.

## Chapter 7 – The Unthinkable Happens – Second Attack

I'm the gardener at my home. In July 2008, all our gardens needed mulch, especially a new shade garden under our maple. So my husband brought home a trailer load of mulch. Mulch can be messy so I slipped on an old pair of running shoes. I had transferred the arch support inserts from these old shoes into my new running shoes. Big mistake going without those inserts, however I didn't even think about it at the time.

To spread the mulch, I'd load up the wheelbarrow and roll it over to the garden. Then shovel out the mulch and spread it around. I was stretching, standing at angles on the hill and the garden edge to spread it evenly without crushing it. It was a tough job. I finally finished after six hours and hit the shower.

We had a barbecue to attend that evening. One of my friends was telling me about her husband's foot injury.

Yup, you guessed it, plantar fasciitis. He was wearing some new, very expensive running shoes and hobbling around. My right foot seemed to be bothering me a bit but I thought it was just in empathy.

Wrong. For several weeks, I was in denial that there was anything wrong with my right foot. After all, it was my left foot that had plantar fasciitis previously. This time wasn't as bad as the first injury. I now know that the acute pain I experienced with the first injury was a severe tear. This time, the cause was just the excess strain from not wearing my arch supports while carrying extra weight from the wheelbarrow and twisting and turning my foot while spreading the mulch. However, the morning pain was there. It was five years since my previous injury.

I was angry with myself for forgetting about the inserts. I didn't want to wait months to heal like the last time. I was depressed and upset. Little did I know what I was about to discover.

About a year before, I injured my back. A series of chiropractic treatments had resolved the problem. Now I get monthly back adjustments. At each visit Dr.

Jennifer Moore asks how I am. Although it didn't relate to my back, I mentioned my sore foot. 'Oh', she replied matter-of-factly, 'we do feet too. I'll have a look at your foot after we adjust your back.' I was surprised.

She checked my foot and made some adjustments. I had to hang onto the bench as she did pull quite hard. She pushed my toes up, and pulled my foot. It was slightly uncomfortable but not painful. She suggested getting a tennis ball and rolling it under the arch of my foot for a few minutes once or twice a day. Also, I was to stretch my toes before getting up in the morning by curling them under and then stretching them up. This was the first time anyone had mentioned exercises or stretching to treat my foot.

Amazingly, after that one treatment, in 3 days, yes only 3 days, I could get up in the morning with no pain, just a slight discomfort. The pain was reduced by 90%. Within a couple of weeks, I felt my plantar fasciitis injury was completely healed.

The timing of the treatment was ideal. I was vacationing on a cruise in the Caribbean two weeks later. I was able to wear my sandals without any discomfort and enjoy walking on the beach.

When I returned home, I started doing research into chiropractic treatment for plantar fasciitis. I hadn't done research of any kind when I first experienced plantar fasciitis back in the spring of 2003. Yet as I looked back, I realized I'd gotten little information and some inaccurate advice from the so called experts. I wondered if the information about chiropractic treatments was common knowledge and I just didn't know about it. So I searched online and in the forums. There was virtually nothing on the internet or in the forums about it. Why wasn't this information getting out to people suffering from plantar fasciitis?

The following month, at my chiropractic appointment, Dr. Moore checked my foot again and did another minor adjustment. I haven't needed any more since. I could hardly believe that I was healed in basically 72 hours compared to a year and a half for my first injury.

I wondered if I was just lucky to heal so quickly or if this was normal. On my next visit to Dr. Moore, I asked if everyone heals this quickly. 'Pretty much unless they have heel spurs, then it can take a bit longer', she answered. I also questioned why more people didn't get chiropractic treatment for plantar fasciitis. She shrugged and guessed it is was due to chiropractors being associated with resolving issues with the back, neck and shoulders more than foot problems.

Compared to many plantar fasciitis treatments, I found it quite affordable. I pay $33 for a chiropractic session. I had two sessions with adjustments to my foot totaling $66 for complete healing. I paid $75 for the first set of shoe inserts from the foot clinic. To me, that's an incredible value for almost instant relief. Often chiropractic treatments are covered under health insurance. My insurer pays 80% making my portion of the two chiropractic treatments only $13.20!

Getting chiropractic adjustments for plantar fasciitis was a fast resolution. For some reason, this information is not widely known. I encourage you to visit a chiropractor. He or she may be able to provide the relief you are searching for and greatly reduce your time to heal.

## Into the Future with Happy Feet

I sincerely hope this information will be useful to you and get you back on your healthy feet soon.

Once you have recovered from your plantar fasciitis injury, remember to keep up your maintenance to prevent future injuries. Keep wearing your arch supports. Buy well fitting footwear. Reduce your weight if that applies to you. And, continue the stretching exercises as the fasciae lose their elasticity with age.

May you be blessed with happy feet.

*Susan Dumas*

## Dedication

This book is dedicated to Dr. Jennifer Moore, B.Sc. Hon., D.C. for her healing abilities that enabled my swift recovery.

Thank you, Jennifer.

## Resources

Rick Gallop's G.I. Diet website is – www.gidiet.com. He also publishes a book called the G.I. Diet Clinic which you can follow for thirteen weeks as if you were attending a clinic.

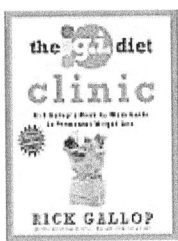

Jorge Cruise's website for the 3-Hour Diet and other resources is – www.jorgecruise.com.

www.ingramcontent.com/pod-product-compliance
Lightning Source LLC
Chambersburg PA
CBHW062110280526
45788CB00003B/1421